GOUT DIET COOKBOOK

FOR SENIORS

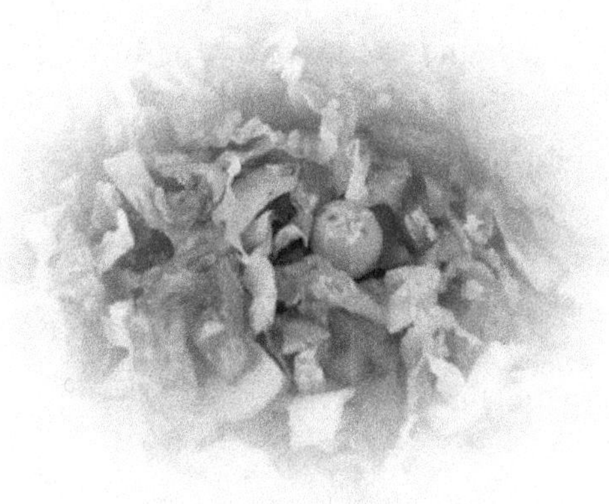

1500-Days Easy, Healthy, And Delicious Recipes To Help Lower Uric Acid Levels, Manage Gout, And Reduce Painful Attacks

Dr. Charlene Alexander

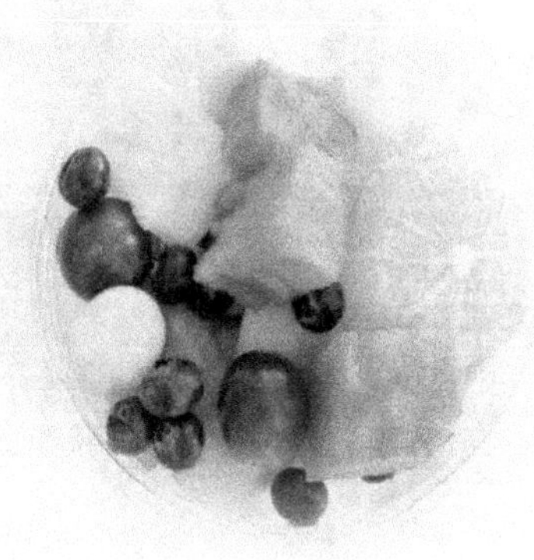

Table of Contents

CHAPTER 5: Snacks and Sides 66

CHAPTER 6: Soups and Salads 76

INTRODUCTION

Welcome to our Gout Diet Cookbook for Seniors, a tailored guide designed to help you navigate the challenges of managing gout through diet and lifestyle adjustments. This cookbook is more than just a collection of recipes; it's a comprehensive resource aimed at enhancing your understanding of gout, its triggers, and how the foods you eat can play a pivotal role in managing symptoms and reducing flare-ups.

Gout, a form of arthritis, can cause significant discomfort and mobility issues, especially in seniors. It's characterized by sudden, severe attacks of pain, redness, and tenderness in joints, often the joint at the base of the big toe. Gout is caused by elevated levels of uric acid in the blood, leading to the formation of urate crystals around joints, which results in inflammation and acute pain.

Diet plays a crucial role in managing gout. Certain foods can raise uric acid levels, while others can help maintain them at a healthier level. Understanding which foods to avoid and which to include in your diet can be a powerful tool in controlling gout symptoms and improving your overall quality of life.

This cookbook is designed with simplicity and practicality in mind, tailored specifically for seniors. It provides easy-to-understand information about gout and its dietary management, tips for meal planning and preparation, and a wide range of recipes that are both delicious and gout-friendly. From hearty breakfasts to nourishing dinners, each recipe is carefully crafted to ensure it meets the dietary needs of those managing gout, without compromising on taste or variety.

We aim to empower you with the knowledge and tools you need to make informed dietary choices that can help manage your gout symptoms. Whether you're new to dietary management of gout or looking for new ideas to add to your meal plan, this cookbook is here to support you on your journey to better health and well-being.

Let's embark on this journey together, to make every meal not just a means to nourish your body, but also a step towards managing your gout more effectively. Welcome to a world of flavors that love you back!

CHAPTER 1: Understanding Gout in Seniors

Gout is a common and complex form of arthritis that can affect anyone, but it has a particular significance in the senior population. Characterized by sudden, severe attacks of pain, swelling, redness, and tenderness in one or more joints, often the base of the big toe, gout can significantly impact the quality of life and mobility of older adults.

The Basics of Gout

Gout occurs when urate crystals accumulate in the joint, causing the inflammation and intense pain of a gout attack. Urate crystals can form when there are high levels of uric acid in the blood. Your body produces uric acid when it breaks down purines — substances that are found naturally in the body as well as in certain foods and beverages. While uric acid is usually dissolved in the blood and passed through the kidneys into the urine, sometimes the body either produces too much uric acid or the kidneys excrete too little. When this happens, uric acid can build up, forming sharp, needle-like urate crystals in a joint or surrounding tissue that cause pain, inflammation, and swelling.

Factors Contributing to Gout in Seniors

Several factors can contribute to the increased risk of developing gout in seniors:

Age and Sex: Men are more likely to develop gout earlier in life, typically between the ages of 30 and 50, whereas women are more likely to develop symptoms after menopause when their uric acid levels approach those of men.

Medical Conditions: Seniors often have other health conditions, such as high blood pressure, diabetes, and kidney disease, which can increase the risk of gout.

Medications: Certain medications that are common among seniors, such as thiazide diuretics (used to treat hypertension) and low-dose aspirin, can also increase uric acid levels.

Diet: A diet rich in meat, seafood, sugary beverages, and alcohol can raise the level of uric acid, leading to gout.

Obesity: Being overweight increases the risk of gout since there is more tissue available for the turnover or breakdown, which leads to more uric acid production.

Symptoms and Diagnosis

Gout symptoms in seniors may sometimes be less typical than in younger individuals. While the classic gout flare involves sudden, intense pain in one joint (often the big toe), seniors might experience a more gradual onset of pain and may have more than one joint affected. Diagnosis typically involves the clinical evaluation of symptoms, blood tests to measure uric acid levels, and sometimes joint fluid tests or imaging studies to confirm the presence of urate crystals.

Management and Treatment

Management of gout in seniors requires a comprehensive approach. It involves not only treating acute gout attacks with medications such as nonsteroidal anti-inflammatory drugs (NSAIDs), colchicine, or corticosteroids but also long-term management strategies to reduce uric acid levels and prevent future attacks. Lifestyle and dietary changes play a crucial role in this long-term management, aiming to reduce the intake of purine-rich foods, alcohol, and sugary drinks while encouraging hydration and a balanced diet rich in fruits, vegetables, whole grains, and low-fat dairy products.

Understanding gout in seniors is crucial for effective management and improving quality of life. Through a combination of medical treatment and lifestyle modifications, including dietary changes as outlined in this cookbook, seniors can manage their gout symptoms more effectively and maintain their mobility and independence.

The Role of Diet in Managing Gout

Diet plays a significant role in the management of gout, a form of arthritis characterized by painful flare-ups in the joints. While medication is essential for acute attacks and long-term control of uric acid levels, dietary choices can greatly influence the frequency and severity of gout attacks. Understanding the relationship between diet and gout is key to minimizing symptoms and improving overall health.

Impact of Diet on Uric Acid Levels

Gout is directly related to the levels of uric acid in the blood. When these levels become too high, uric acid can form crystals in and around the joints, leading to inflammation, pain, and swelling. Diet influences uric acid levels, with certain foods and beverages either exacerbating or alleviating the condition.

Foods to Avoid

High-Purine Foods: Purines are naturally occurring substances found in various foods. During digestion, purines are broken down into uric acid. Foods high in purines, such as red meat, organ meats (like liver and kidneys), and certain types of seafood (such as anchovies, sardines, mussels, and scallops), can raise uric acid levels and should be consumed in moderation or avoided.

Sugary Foods and Beverages: Foods and drinks high in fructose and sucrose can increase uric acid levels. This includes sugary sodas, candies, and desserts.

Alcohol: Alcohol consumption, especially beer and spirits, can interfere with the elimination of uric acid from the body, leading to higher levels in the blood.

Foods to Include

Low-Purine Choices: Eating more low-purine foods can help manage gout. These include fruits, vegetables, whole grains, and most dairy products, especially low-fat options.

Cherries and Vitamin C: Some studies suggest that cherries and cherry juice can reduce gout flare-ups due to their antioxidant properties. Similarly, foods rich in vitamin C like oranges, strawberries, and bell peppers may help lower uric acid levels.

Water and Hydration: Staying well-hydrated is crucial for people with gout, as water can help flush uric acid from the body and reduce the risk of crystal formation.

Dietary Strategies

Weight Management: Maintaining a healthy weight can reduce the risk of gout attacks. Excess weight can increase uric acid levels and put more stress on the joints.

Balanced Diet: Adopting a balanced diet rich in fruits, vegetables, whole grains, and lean proteins can support overall health and help manage gout.

Moderation: It's essential to consume high-purine foods and alcohol in moderation, focusing instead on a diet that supports overall well-being and gout management.

The Big Picture

Diet is not a standalone cure for gout but an integral part of a comprehensive management plan. It works alongside medication and lifestyle changes to help reduce the frequency and severity of gout attacks. By making informed dietary choices, individuals with gout can take proactive steps toward managing their condition and improving their quality of life. This cookbook aims to provide delicious, gout-friendly recipes that align with these dietary principles, making it easier for seniors to enjoy a diverse and nutritious diet while managing gout.

The Importance of Hydration in Managing Gout

Hydration plays a crucial role in the management and prevention of gout, a condition characterized by painful flare-ups in the joints due to the accumulation of uric acid crystals. Adequate fluid intake is essential for everyone, but it becomes even more critical for individuals with gout. Here's why staying hydrated is vital for those managing this condition:

1. Uric Acid Dilution

Water helps dilute the concentrations of uric acid in the bloodstream. By increasing the volume of urine, water facilitates the excretion of uric acid, reducing the likelihood of crystal formation in the joints. Drinking plenty of fluids can thus be seen as a natural way to flush excess uric acid out of the body.

2. Prevention of Kidney Stones

Individuals with gout are at an increased risk of developing kidney stones, which can occur when uric acid accumulates in the kidneys. Adequate hydration can prevent the formation of these stones by keeping the kidneys flushed and reducing the concentration of uric acid in the urine.

3. Improved Kidney Function

Good hydration supports overall kidney function, which is vital for the elimination of waste products, including uric acid. When the body is well-hydrated, the kidneys can more efficiently filter and eliminate toxins, thereby maintaining a healthy balance of uric acid.

4. Reduction in Gout Attacks

Staying hydrated may help reduce the frequency of gout attacks. Adequate fluid intake ensures that uric acid levels are more likely to stay within a manageable range, thereby lowering the risk of sudden and painful gout flare-ups.

Hydration Tips for Gout Management

Aim for 8-12 Cups Daily: The general recommendation is to drink at least eight 8-ounce glasses of fluids a day, but individuals with gout may benefit from slightly more, depending on their specific needs and lifestyle factors.

Water is Best: Pure water is the most effective hydrator and should constitute the majority of your fluid intake. It's calorie-free, caffeine-free, and doesn't contain any substances that might raise uric acid levels.

Monitor Your Urine: The color of your urine can be a good indicator of hydration status. Aim for light yellow; dark urine can be a sign of dehydration.

Incorporate Hydrating Foods: Fruits and vegetables with high water content, such as cucumbers, tomatoes, watermelon, and oranges, can contribute to your overall fluid intake.

Limit Dehydrating Beverages: While staying hydrated, it's also important to limit or avoid alcohol and beverages high in caffeine, as these can dehydrate the body and exacerbate gout symptoms.

CHAPTER 2: Breakfast Recipes

Banana and Walnut Smoothie

Ingredients:

- 1 ripe banana, peeled and sliced
- 1/4 cup walnuts
- 1 cup almond milk or preferred non-dairy milk
- 1/2 teaspoon vanilla extract
- Ice cubes (optional)
- A pinch of cinnamon (optional)

Instructions:

1. Combine the banana, walnuts, almond milk, and vanilla extract in a blender. Add ice cubes if you like your smoothie cold.
2. Blend until smooth. Add more almond milk if needed to adjust the consistency.
3. Pour into a glass, sprinkle with a pinch of cinnamon, and enjoy immediately.

Avocado Toast on Whole Grain Bread

Ingredients:

- 1 ripe avocado
- 2 slices of whole-grain bread
- Salt and pepper to taste

- Red pepper flakes (optional)

- A squeeze of lemon juice (optional)

- Fresh herbs like parsley or chives for garnish (optional)

Instructions:

1. Toast the whole-grain bread slices to your preferred level of crispiness.

2. In a bowl, mash the ripe avocado with a fork until it reaches a smooth consistency. Season with salt, pepper, and lemon juice to taste.

3. Spread the mashed avocado evenly over the toasted bread slices.

4. If desired, sprinkle with red pepper flakes and garnish with fresh herbs.

5. Serve immediately and enjoy a healthy, nutritious start to your day.

Quinoa Breakfast Bowl

Ingredients:

- 1 cup cooked quinoa

- 1/2 cup fresh berries (such as blueberries, raspberries, or strawberries)

- 1/4 cup sliced almonds or chopped walnuts

- 1 tablespoon chia seeds

- Honey or maple syrup to taste

- Almond milk or preferred non-dairy milk, for serving

Instructions:

1. Start with cooked quinoa as the base of your bowl. Ensure the quinoa is fluffed and cooled slightly.
2. Add the fresh berries on top of the quinoa for a burst of flavor and antioxidants.
3. Sprinkle the sliced almonds or chopped walnuts over the berries for a crunchy texture and healthy fats.
4. Add chia seeds for an extra nutritional boost, including fiber and omega-3 fatty acids.
5. Drizzle honey or maple syrup over the bowl for a touch of natural sweetness.
6. Pour a bit of almond milk around the edges of the bowl, allowing you to mix everything for a creamy consistency.
7. Mix all the ingredients just before eating, and enjoy a nutritious and delicious start to your day.

Apple Cinnamon Porridge

Ingredients:

- 1 cup rolled oats
- 2 cups water or non-dairy milk
- 1 medium apple, peeled and diced
- 1/2 teaspoon ground cinnamon

- 1 tablespoon maple syrup or honey

- A pinch of salt

- Chopped nuts or seeds for topping (optional)

Instructions:

1. In a medium saucepan, bring the water or non-dairy milk to a boil. Add a pinch of salt.

2. Stir in the rolled oats and reduce the heat to a simmer. Cook the oats, stirring occasionally, until they begin to soften.

3. Add the diced apple and ground cinnamon to the saucepan. Continue to cook the mixture, stirring occasionally, until the oats are fully cooked and the apple pieces are tender.

4. Sweeten the porridge with maple syrup or honey, adjusting the amount to suit your taste.

5. Serve the porridge in bowls, and if desired, top with chopped nuts or seeds for added texture and nutrition.

6. Enjoy your warm and comforting apple cinnamon porridge, perfect for a cozy morning.

Vegetable Omelet

Ingredients:

- 2 large eggs

- 1/4 cup diced vegetables (such as bell peppers, onions, spinach, and mushrooms)

- Salt and pepper to taste

- 1 teaspoon olive oil

- Shredded cheese (optional, choose low-fat)

Instructions:

1. Beat the eggs in a bowl, and season with salt and pepper.

2. Heat olive oil in a non-stick skillet over medium heat.

3. Sauté the diced vegetables in the skillet until they are soft and lightly browned.

4. Pour the beaten eggs over the vegetables, tilting the pan to spread them evenly.

5. Cook until the eggs are set on the bottom, then use a spatula to gently fold the omelet in half.

6. Cook for another minute, or until the omelet is fully set.

7. Serve hot, garnished with a sprinkle of shredded cheese if desired.

Whole Wheat Pancakes with Maple Syrup

Ingredients:

- 1 cup whole wheat flour

- 1 tablespoon sugar (optional)

- 2 teaspoons baking powder

- 1/2 teaspoon salt

- 1 egg, beaten

- 1 cup non-dairy milk

- 2 tablespoons unsweetened applesauce or melted coconut oil

- Pure maple syrup for serving

Instructions:

1. In a large bowl, whisk together the whole wheat flour, sugar (if using), baking powder, and salt.

2. In another bowl, combine the beaten egg, non-dairy milk, and applesauce or melted coconut oil.

3. Pour the wet ingredients into the dry ingredients and stir until just combined; the batter may be slightly lumpy.

4. Heat a non-stick skillet or griddle over medium heat and lightly coat with cooking spray or a dab of oil.

5. Pour 1/4 cup of batter for each pancake onto the skillet. Cook until bubbles form on the surface, then flip and cook until golden brown on the other side.

6. Serve the pancakes hot, drizzled with pure maple syrup.

Chia Seed Pudding with Kiwi

Ingredients:

- 1/4 cup chia seeds

- 1 cup almond milk or any non-dairy milk of choice

- 1-2 tablespoons honey or maple syrup (adjust to taste)

- 1/2 teaspoon vanilla extract (optional)

- 2 ripe kiwis, peeled and sliced

Instructions:

1. In a mixing bowl, combine the chia seeds with almond milk. Stir well to prevent clumping.
2. Add honey or maple syrup and vanilla extract to the mixture, blending thoroughly.
3. Cover the bowl and refrigerate for at least 2 hours or overnight, allowing the chia seeds to absorb the liquid and swell, forming a pudding-like consistency.
4. Before serving, stir the pudding to ensure it's well-mixed. If it's too thick, you can add a little more almond milk to reach your desired consistency.
5. Serve the chia pudding in bowls or glasses, layered or topped with fresh kiwi slices.

Cottage Cheese with Pineapple

Ingredients:

- 1 cup low-fat cottage cheese
- 1/2 cup fresh pineapple chunks or rings (canned in juice, not syrup, can be used if drained well)
- A sprinkle of cinnamon or nutmeg (optional)

Instructions:

1. Place the cottage cheese in a serving bowl.
2. Top the cottage cheese with fresh pineapple chunks or arrange pineapple rings neatly on top.
3. For added flavor, sprinkle a dash of cinnamon or nutmeg over the pineapple and cottage cheese.
4. Serve immediately.

Almond Butter and Banana Sandwich

Ingredients:

- 2 slices of whole-grain bread
- 2 tablespoons almond butter
- 1 ripe banana, sliced
- A sprinkle of cinnamon (optional)

Instructions:

1. Toast the whole-grain bread slices to your desired level of crispiness.
2. Spread almond butter evenly on one side of each toasted bread slice.
3. Arrange the sliced banana on top of one of the almond butter-covered slices.
4. If desired, sprinkle a little cinnamon over the banana slices for added flavor.

5. Place the other slice of bread, almond butter side down, on top
    of the bananas to form a sandwich.

6. Cut the sandwich in half and serve immediately.

Veggie Breakfast Wrap

Ingredients:

- 1 whole wheat or low-carb tortilla

- 2 eggs (or egg whites for a lower-fat option)

- 1/4 cup diced vegetables (such as bell peppers, onions, spinach,
  and mushrooms)

- 1 tablespoon shredded low-fat cheese (optional)

- Salt and pepper to taste

- 1 teaspoon olive oil

Instructions:

1. Heat the olive oil in a non-stick skillet over medium heat.

2. Add the diced vegetables to the skillet and sauté until they are
    soft and lightly browned.

3. Beat the eggs in a bowl, season with salt and pepper, and add
    them to the skillet with the vegetables. Stir gently to scramble
    the eggs with the veggies.

4. Warm the tortilla in a separate skillet or microwave for a few
    seconds to make it pliable.

5. Place the cooked veggie and egg mixture in the center of the tortilla. Sprinkle with shredded cheese if using.

6. Fold the bottom of the tortilla over the filling, then fold in the sides and roll up tightly.

7. Serve the wrap immediately, cut in half if desired.

Baked Sweet Potato Hash

Ingredients:

- 2 large sweet potatoes, peeled and diced
- 1 bell pepper, diced
- 1 medium onion, diced
- 2 tablespoons olive oil
- Salt and pepper to taste
- Fresh herbs (like thyme or rosemary), finely chopped (optional)

Instructions:

1. Preheat the oven to 400°F (200°C).

2. In a large bowl, toss the diced sweet potatoes, bell pepper, and onion with olive oil until evenly coated. Season with salt, pepper, and if desired, some finely chopped fresh herbs.

3. Spread the vegetable mixture in a single layer on a baking sheet lined with parchment paper.

4. Bake in the preheated oven for about 25-30 minutes, or until the sweet potatoes are tender and lightly browned, stirring halfway through the cooking time.

5. Serve the sweet potato hash warm.

Pear and Ginger Muffins

Ingredients:

- 2 cups whole wheat flour
- 1/2 cup sugar or preferred sweetener
- 2 teaspoons baking powder
- 1/2 teaspoon baking soda
- 1/4 teaspoon salt
- 1 tablespoon ground ginger
- 1/2 teaspoon cinnamon
- 2 ripe pears, peeled, cored, and diced
- 2 large eggs
- 1/4 cup unsweetened applesauce
- 1/4 cup vegetable oil
- 1/2 cup non-dairy milk
- 1 teaspoon vanilla extract

Instructions:

1. Preheat the oven to 375°F (190°C) and line a muffin tin with paper liners or lightly grease it.

2. In a large bowl, whisk together the whole wheat flour, sugar, baking powder, baking soda, salt, ground ginger, and cinnamon.

3. In a separate bowl, beat the eggs, and then mix in the applesauce, vegetable oil, non-dairy milk, and vanilla extract.

4. Add the wet ingredients to the dry ingredients, stirring just until combined. Fold in the diced pears gently.

5. Spoon the batter into the prepared muffin tin, filling each cup about 3/4 full.

6. Bake for 18-20 minutes, or until a toothpick inserted into the center of a muffin comes out clean.

7. Allow the muffins to cool in the pan for a few minutes before transferring them to a wire rack to cool completely.

8. Serve and enjoy the pear and ginger muffins.

Grilled Chicken Salad with Mixed Greens

Ingredients:

- 1 boneless, skinless chicken breast
- Salt and pepper to taste
- Mixed salad greens (lettuce, spinach, arugula, etc.)
- Cherry tomatoes, halved
- Cucumber, sliced
- Red onion, thinly sliced
- Olive oil
- Balsamic vinegar or lemon juice

Instructions:

1. Preheat the grill to medium-high heat. Season the chicken breast with salt and pepper.
2. Grill the chicken for 6-7 minutes on each side or until fully cooked and the internal temperature reaches 165°F (74°C). Let it rest for a few minutes, then slice thinly.
3. In a large salad bowl, combine the mixed greens, cherry tomatoes, cucumber slices, and red onion.
4. Drizzle olive oil and balsamic vinegar or lemon juice over the salad, and toss gently to coat.
5. Arrange the grilled chicken slices on top of the salad.

6. Serve immediately, offering additional dressing on the side if desired.

Quinoa and Black Bean Stuffed Peppers

Ingredients:

- 4 large bell peppers, any color

- 1 cup cooked quinoa

- 1 can (15 oz) black beans, rinsed and drained

- 1 cup corn kernels (fresh, canned, or thawed from frozen)

- 1/2 cup diced tomatoes (fresh or canned without added salt)

- 1 teaspoon cumin

- 1 teaspoon paprika

- Salt and pepper to taste

- Shredded low-fat cheese (optional)

- Fresh cilantro, chopped (for garnish)

Instructions:

1. Preheat the oven to 350°F (175°C). Slice the tops off the bell peppers and remove the seeds and membranes.

2. In a bowl, mix the cooked quinoa, black beans, corn, and diced tomatoes. Season with cumin, paprika, salt, and pepper.

3. Stuff each bell pepper with the quinoa mixture, packing it down to fit as much as possible.

4. Place the stuffed peppers upright in a baking dish. Add a small amount of water to the bottom of the dish to prevent sticking and help steam the peppers.

5. Cover with foil and bake for about 30-35 minutes, or until the peppers are tender.

6. If using cheese, sprinkle it over the top of each pepper during the last 5 minutes of baking, and return to the oven uncovered until the cheese is melted.

7. Garnish with fresh cilantro before serving.

Lentil Soup with Carrots and Celery

Ingredients:

- 1 cup dried lentils, rinsed and drained
- 1 tablespoon olive oil
- 1 onion, chopped
- 2 carrots, peeled and diced
- 2 stalks celery, diced
- 2 cloves garlic, minced
- 4 cups vegetable broth or water
- 1 teaspoon ground cumin
- Salt and pepper to taste
- Fresh parsley, chopped (for garnish)

Instructions:

1. Heat olive oil in a large pot over medium heat. Add the chopped onion, carrots, and celery. Sauté until the vegetables are softened, about 5 minutes.

2. Add the minced garlic and sauté for another minute until fragrant.

3. Stir in the lentils, vegetable broth, and cumin. Season with salt and pepper.

4. Bring the mixture to a boil, then reduce the heat to low, cover, and simmer for about 25-30 minutes, or until the lentils are tender.

5. Taste and adjust the seasoning if necessary. You can blend a portion of the soup for a creamier texture if desired.

6. Serve hot, garnished with fresh parsley.

Turkey and Avocado Wrap

Ingredients:

- 1 whole wheat tortilla or wrap
- 2-3 slices of deli turkey breast (low-sodium)
- 1/2 ripe avocado, sliced
- Lettuce leaves
- Sliced tomato
- 1 tablespoon mustard or hummus

- Salt and pepper to taste

Instructions:

1. Lay the whole wheat tortilla flat on a plate or cutting board.
2. Spread mustard or hummus evenly over the tortilla.
3. Arrange the lettuce leaves in the center of the tortilla, leaving space around the edges for folding.
4. Place the turkey slices on top of the lettuce. Add the sliced avocado and tomato on top of the turkey.
5. Season with a pinch of salt and pepper.
6. To wrap, fold in the sides of the tortilla first, then roll it up from the bottom, tucking in the fillings as you go.
7. Cut the wrap in half diagonally and serve immediately.

Roasted Beet and Goat Cheese Salad

Ingredients:

- 4 medium beets, scrubbed, trimmed, and cut into wedges
- 2 tablespoons olive oil
- Salt and pepper to taste
- Mixed salad greens (such as arugula, spinach, or lettuce)
- 1/4 cup goat cheese, crumbled
- 1/4 cup walnuts, toasted and chopped
- Balsamic vinegar or balsamic glaze for dressing

Instructions:

1. Preheat your oven to 400°F (200°C). Toss the beet wedges with olive oil, salt, and pepper in a bowl.

2. Spread the beets on a baking sheet in a single layer. Roast in the preheated oven for 25-30 minutes or until beets are tender and slightly caramelized, stirring halfway through.

3. Allow the roasted beets to cool slightly.

4. Arrange the mixed salad greens on a serving platter or individual plates. Top with the roasted beets, crumbled goat cheese, and toasted walnuts.

5. Drizzle with balsamic vinegar or balsamic glaze just before serving.

Tofu Stir-Fry with Broccoli and Bell Peppers

Ingredients:

- 1 block (14 oz) firm tofu, drained and cut into cubes
- 2 tablespoons soy sauce or tamari
- 1 tablespoon sesame oil
- 1 tablespoon vegetable oil
- 1 head of broccoli, cut into florets
- 1 bell pepper, sliced
- 2 cloves garlic, minced

- 1 teaspoon fresh ginger, grated

- 2 green onions, sliced for garnish

- Sesame seeds for garnish (optional)

Instructions:

1. Press the tofu to remove excess moisture, then cut into cubes. Toss the tofu cubes with soy sauce and let marinate for at least 10 minutes.

2. Heat the sesame oil and vegetable oil in a large skillet or wok over medium-high heat. Add the tofu cubes and stir-fry until golden brown on all sides. Remove tofu from the skillet and set aside.

3. In the same skillet, add the broccoli florets and bell pepper slices. Stir-fry for 4-5 minutes, or until the vegetables are tender-crisp.

4. Add the minced garlic and grated ginger to the skillet with the vegetables and stir-fry for an additional minute until fragrant.

5. Return the tofu to the skillet with the vegetables. Toss everything together and heat through.

6. Serve the tofu stir-fry garnished with sliced green onions and sesame seeds if desired.

Egg Salad on Whole Grain Bread

Ingredients:

- 4 hard-boiled eggs, peeled and chopped

- 2 tablespoons low-fat Greek yogurt

- 1 tablespoon Dijon mustard

- Salt and pepper to taste

- 1/4 cup finely chopped celery

- 1/4 cup finely chopped red onion

- 4 slices of whole-grain bread

- Lettuce leaves (optional)

- Sliced tomatoes (optional)

Instructions:

1. In a bowl, combine the chopped hard-boiled eggs, Greek yogurt, and Dijon mustard. Mix well.

2. Season the egg mixture with salt and pepper to taste.

3. Fold in the finely chopped celery and red onion until evenly distributed.

4. Toast the whole grain bread slices if desired.

5. Spread the egg salad evenly over two slices of the toasted whole-grain bread.

6. Add lettuce and tomato slices if using, then top with the remaining slices of bread to form sandwiches.

7. Cut the sandwiches in half and serve immediately for a nutritious and satisfying lunch.

Vegetable and Chickpea Curry

Ingredients:

- 1 tablespoon vegetable oil
- 1 onion, finely chopped
- 2 cloves garlic, minced
- 1 tablespoon curry powder (adjust according to taste)
- 1 can (15 oz) chickpeas, rinsed and drained
- 1 can (14.5 oz) diced tomatoes, undrained
- 1 cup cauliflower florets
- 1 cup diced carrots
- 1 cup diced potatoes
- 1 can (13.5 oz) coconut milk
- Salt to taste
- Fresh cilantro, chopped (for garnish)
- Cooked rice or naan bread, for serving

Instructions:

1. Heat the vegetable oil in a large pan over medium heat. Add the chopped onion and sauté until soft and translucent.
2. Add the minced garlic and curry powder to the pan, stirring well for about 1 minute until fragrant.

3. Stir in the chickpeas, diced tomatoes (with their juice), cauliflower florets, diced carrots, and diced potatoes. Mix well to ensure the vegetables are coated with the curry mixture.

4. Pour in the coconut milk and stir to combine. Bring the mixture to a simmer.

5. Reduce the heat to low, cover the pan, and let the curry cook for about 20-25 minutes, or until the vegetables are tender.

6. Season the curry with salt to taste.

7. Serve the vegetable and chickpea curry garnished with chopped cilantro, accompanied by cooked rice or naan bread.

Baked Salmon with Dill and Lemon

Ingredients:

- 4 salmon fillets (about 6 ounces each)
- 2 tablespoons olive oil
- Salt and pepper to taste
- 2 teaspoons fresh dill, chopped (or 1 teaspoon dried dill)
- 1 lemon, thinly sliced
- Additional lemon wedges for serving

Instructions:

1. Preheat your oven to 400°F (200°C). Line a baking sheet with parchment paper or lightly grease it.

2. Place the salmon fillets on the prepared baking sheet. Drizzle each fillet with olive oil and rub it over the surface.

3. Season the salmon with salt and pepper. Sprinkle the chopped dill evenly over each fillet.

4. Arrange lemon slices on top of the salmon fillets, covering them as much as possible.

5. Bake in the preheated oven for 12-15 minutes or until the salmon flakes easily with a fork.

6. Serve the baked salmon immediately, with additional lemon wedges on the side for squeezing over the fish.

Pasta Primavera with Olive Oil and Garlic

Ingredients:

- 12 ounces whole wheat pasta (such as spaghetti or fettuccine)
- 1/4 cup olive oil
- 4 cloves garlic, minced
- 1 cup broccoli florets
- 1 cup sliced bell peppers (any color)
- 1 cup cherry tomatoes, halved
- 1/2 cup carrots, julienned
- 1/2 cup peas (fresh or frozen)
- Salt and pepper to taste
- Freshly grated Parmesan cheese (optional)
- Fresh basil leaves, torn (for garnish)

Instructions:

1. Cook the pasta according to package instructions in a large pot of boiling salted water until al dente. Drain and set aside, reserving some pasta water.

2. While the pasta cooks, heat the olive oil in a large skillet over medium heat. Add the minced garlic and sauté for 1-2 minutes until fragrant but not browned.

3. Add the broccoli, bell peppers, cherry tomatoes, carrots, and peas to the skillet. Sauté the vegetables, stirring occasionally, until they are tender but still crisp, about 5-7 minutes.

4. Add the cooked pasta to the skillet with the vegetables. Toss well to combine, adding a splash of reserved pasta water if needed to loosen the sauce.

5. Season the pasta primavera with salt and pepper to taste. Serve hot, garnished with freshly grated Parmesan cheese (if using) and torn fresh basil leaves.

Zucchini Noodles with Tomato and Basil Sauce

Ingredients:

- 4 medium zucchinis
- 2 tablespoons olive oil
- 2 cloves garlic, minced
- 1 can (14 oz) diced tomatoes, undrained

- Salt and pepper to taste

- 1/2 teaspoon dried oregano (optional)

- Fresh basil leaves, chopped

- Grated Parmesan cheese (optional, for serving)

Instructions:

1. Use a spiralizer to turn the zucchini into noodles. Set aside.

2. Heat 1 tablespoon of olive oil in a large skillet over medium heat. Add the minced garlic and sauté for about 1 minute until fragrant.

3. Add the diced tomatoes (with their juice) to the skillet. Season with salt, pepper, and dried oregano if using. Simmer the sauce for about 10-15 minutes until it thickens slightly.

4. In another skillet, heat the remaining tablespoon of olive oil over medium heat. Add the zucchini noodles and sauté for 2-3 minutes until just tender. Be careful not to overcook to avoid the noodles becoming mushy.

5. Serve the zucchini noodles topped with the tomato and basil sauce. Garnish with fresh basil and grated Parmesan cheese if desired.

Spinach and Feta Stuffed Chicken Breast

Ingredients:

- 4 boneless, skinless chicken breasts

- Salt and pepper to taste

- 1 cup fresh spinach, chopped

- 1/2 cup feta cheese, crumbled

- 2 tablespoons olive oil

- 1 clove garlic, minced

- Toothpicks (for securing)

Instructions:

1. Preheat your oven to 375°F (190°C).

2. Make a horizontal cut along the side of each chicken breast to create a pocket, being careful not to cut all the way through.

3. Season the inside and outside of the chicken breasts with salt and pepper.

4. In a bowl, mix the chopped spinach, crumbled feta cheese, and minced garlic.

5. Stuff each chicken breast with the spinach and feta mixture, then secure the open side with toothpicks.

6. Heat olive oil in an ovenproof skillet over medium-high heat. Sear the stuffed chicken breasts for 2-3 minutes on each side until golden brown.

7. Transfer the skillet to the preheated oven and bake for 20-25 minutes, or until the chicken is cooked through and no longer pink in the center.

8. Remove the toothpicks before serving. Enjoy the stuffed chicken breasts with a side of your choice, such as roasted vegetables or a garden salad.

Cauliflower Rice Stir-Fry with Mixed Vegetables

Ingredients:

- 1 head of cauliflower, grated or processed into rice-sized pieces
- 2 tablespoons olive oil
- 1 cup mixed vegetables (such as carrots, peas, bell peppers, and broccoli), diced
- 2 cloves garlic, minced
- 1 tablespoon soy sauce or tamari (adjust to taste)
- Salt and pepper to taste
- Green onions, sliced for garnish
- Sesame seeds for garnish (optional)

Instructions:

1. Heat olive oil in a large skillet or wok over medium-high heat.
2. Add the minced garlic and sauté for about 30 seconds until fragrant.
3. Add the mixed vegetables to the skillet and stir-fry for 5-7 minutes until they start to soften.
4. Stir in the cauliflower rice, mixing well with the vegetables.

5. Pour the soy sauce or tamari over the cauliflower rice mixture, stirring to combine. Season with salt and pepper to taste.

6. Continue to stir-fry for an additional 5-8 minutes, or until the cauliflower rice is tender but not mushy.

7. Serve the cauliflower rice stir-fry garnished with sliced green onions and sesame seeds if desired.

Greek Salad with Chickpeas

Ingredients:

- 1 can (15 oz) chickpeas, rinsed and drained
- 2 cups cherry tomatoes, halved
- 1 cucumber, diced
- 1 bell pepper, diced
- 1/2 red onion, thinly sliced
- 1/2 cup Kalamata olives, pitted
- 1/2 cup feta cheese, crumbled
- 2 tablespoons olive oil
- 1 tablespoon red wine vinegar
- 1 teaspoon dried oregano
- Salt and pepper to taste
- Fresh parsley, chopped for garnish

Instructions:

1. In a large salad bowl, combine the rinsed and drained chickpeas, cherry tomatoes, cucumber, bell pepper, red onion, and Kalamata olives.
2. Sprinkle the crumbled feta cheese over the top of the salad.
3. In a small bowl, whisk together the olive oil, red wine vinegar, dried oregano, salt, and pepper to create the dressing.
4. Pour the dressing over the salad and toss gently to ensure all ingredients are well coated.
5. Garnish the Greek salad with chopped fresh parsley before serving. Enjoy this refreshing and protein-packed salad as a nutritious lunch or side dish.

CHAPTER 4: Dinner Recipes

Baked Cod with Lemon and Herbs

Ingredients:

- 4 cod fillets (about 6 ounces each)
- 2 tablespoons olive oil
- Salt and pepper to taste
- 1 lemon, thinly sliced
- 2 tablespoons fresh parsley, chopped
- 2 teaspoons fresh thyme leaves (or 1 teaspoon dried thyme)
- 2 cloves garlic, minced

Instructions:

1. Preheat your oven to 400°F (200°C). Line a baking sheet with parchment paper for easy cleanup.
2. Pat the cod fillets dry with paper towels to remove excess moisture. This helps in getting a nicer sear on the fish.
3. Arrange the cod fillets on the prepared baking sheet. Drizzle olive oil over each fillet, and season with salt and pepper.
4. Place a few lemon slices on top of each fillet. Sprinkle the minced garlic, chopped parsley, and thyme leaves evenly over the fillets.
5. Bake in the preheated oven for 12-15 minutes, or until the fish flakes easily with a fork and is opaque throughout.

6. Serve the baked cod immediately, garnished with additional fresh herbs if desired.

Stuffed Acorn Squash

Ingredients:

- 2 acorn squash, halved and seeds removed
- 1 tablespoon olive oil
- Salt and pepper to taste
- 1 cup quinoa, cooked
- 1/2 cup dried cranberries
- 1/2 cup pecans, chopped
- 2 tablespoons maple syrup
- 1 teaspoon cinnamon
- 1/4 teaspoon nutmeg
- Fresh parsley, chopped for garnish

Instructions:

1. Preheat your oven to 375°F (190°C). Line a baking sheet with parchment paper.
2. Brush the cut sides of the acorn squash with olive oil and season with salt and pepper. Place the squash halves cut side down on the prepared baking sheet.
3. Roast the squash in the preheated oven for about 25-30 minutes, or until tender when pierced with a fork.

4. While the squash is roasting, mix the cooked quinoa, dried cranberries, chopped pecans, maple syrup, cinnamon, and nutmeg in a bowl.

5. Once the squash is tender, remove it from the oven and flip the halves so they are cut side up. Spoon the quinoa mixture into the center of each squash half.

6. Return the stuffed squash to the oven and bake for an additional 10-15 minutes, until the filling is heated through.

7. Garnish with chopped parsley before serving. Enjoy this wholesome and flavorful dish as a main course or a hearty side.

Grilled Vegetable Platter

Ingredients:

- 1 zucchini, sliced lengthwise
- 1 yellow squash, sliced lengthwise
- 1 red bell pepper, seeded and quartered
- 1 yellow bell pepper, seeded and quartered
- 1 eggplant, sliced into rounds
- 1 red onion, cut into wedges
- Olive oil for brushing
- Salt and pepper to taste
- Balsamic vinegar (optional for drizzling)
- Fresh herbs like basil or parsley, for garnish

Instructions:

1. Preheat the grill to medium-high heat.

2. Brush the vegetable slices and wedges with olive oil and season them with salt and pepper.

3. Place the vegetables on the grill, working in batches if necessary. Grill each side for about 3-4 minutes or until the vegetables have nice grill marks and are tender.

4. As the vegetables are grilled, transfer them to a serving platter.

5. Once all the vegetables are grilled and arranged on the platter, you can drizzle them with a bit of balsamic vinegar if desired for added flavor.

6. Garnish the platter with fresh herbs before serving.

Lemon Garlic Shrimp and Asparagus

Ingredients:

- 1 pound large shrimp, peeled and deveined
- 1 bunch asparagus, ends trimmed
- 3 tablespoons olive oil
- 3 cloves garlic, minced
- Zest and juice of 1 lemon
- Salt and pepper to taste
- Red pepper flakes (optional, for heat)
- Fresh parsley, chopped for garnish

Instructions:

1. Preheat the grill to medium-high heat.

2. In a large bowl, toss the shrimp and asparagus with olive oil, minced garlic, lemon zest, and lemon juice. Season with salt, pepper, and red pepper flakes if using.

3. Let the mixture marinate for about 10-15 minutes to enhance the flavors.

4. Thread the shrimp onto skewers (if using wooden skewers, soak them in water for at least 30 minutes beforehand to prevent burning).

5. Place the shrimp skewers and asparagus spears directly on the grill.

6. Grill the shrimp for 2-3 minutes on each side or until they turn pink and opaque. Grill the asparagus for 3-4 minutes, turning occasionally, until tender and charred.

7. Transfer the grilled shrimp and asparagus to a serving platter.

8. Garnish with fresh parsley and serve immediately, offering additional lemon wedges on the side if desired.

Roasted Chicken with Root Vegetables

Ingredients:

- 4 chicken thighs (bone-in, skin-on)
- 2 carrots, peeled and cut into chunks

- 2 parsnips, peeled and cut into chunks
- 1 sweet potato, peeled and cut into chunks
- 1 onion, quartered
- 3 tablespoons olive oil
- 2 teaspoons fresh thyme leaves (or 1 teaspoon dried thyme)
- Salt and pepper to taste
- 2 cloves garlic, minced

Instructions:

1. Preheat your oven to 400°F (200°C).
2. In a large bowl, toss the carrots, parsnips, sweet potato, and onion with 2 tablespoons of olive oil, half of the thyme, salt, and pepper.
3. Spread the vegetables in a single layer on a large baking sheet.
4. In the same bowl, mix the chicken thighs with the remaining olive oil, thyme, salt, pepper, and minced garlic, ensuring they are well coated.
5. Place the chicken thighs on top of the vegetables.
6. Roast in the preheated oven for about 45-50 minutes, or until the chicken is cooked through and the vegetables are tender and caramelized.
7. Serve the roasted chicken with the root vegetables, spooning any pan juices over the top.

Vegetarian Chili

Ingredients:

- 2 tablespoons olive oil
- 1 onion, chopped
- 2 bell peppers (any color), chopped
- 2 carrots, peeled and diced
- 2 stalks of celery, diced
- 3 cloves garlic, minced
- 1 can (15 oz) black beans, rinsed and drained
- 1 can (15 oz) kidney beans, rinsed and drained
- 1 can (28 oz) diced tomatoes, undrained
- 2 tablespoons tomato paste
- 1 tablespoon chili powder (adjust to taste)
- 1 teaspoon ground cumin
- 1 teaspoon smoked paprika
- Salt and pepper to taste
- 1 cup vegetable broth (adjust for desired thickness)
- Fresh cilantro, chopped for garnish
- Shredded cheese (optional for serving)

Instructions:

1. Heat the olive oil in a large pot over medium heat.

2. Add the onion, bell peppers, carrots, and celery. Sauté until the vegetables are softened, about 5-7 minutes.

3. Add the minced garlic and cook for another minute until fragrant.

4. Stir in the black beans, kidney beans, diced tomatoes with their juice, tomato paste, chili powder, cumin, smoked paprika, salt, and pepper.

5. Pour in the vegetable broth and stir to combine all the ingredients.

6. Bring the chili to a boil, then reduce the heat to low and simmer, uncovered, for about 30 minutes, stirring occasionally. If the chili is too thick, you can add a little more broth to reach your desired consistency.

7. Taste and adjust the seasoning if necessary.

8. Serve the vegetarian chili hot, garnished with fresh cilantro and shredded cheese if desired.

Mushroom Risotto

Ingredients:

- 1 cup Arborio rice
- 4 cups vegetable broth, warmed
- 1 cup mushrooms, sliced (button, cremini, or a mix)
- 1 small onion, finely chopped
- 2 cloves garlic, minced

- 1/2 cup dry white wine (optional)
- 2 tablespoons olive oil
- 1/4 cup grated Parmesan cheese
- Salt and pepper to taste
- Fresh parsley, chopped for garnish

Instructions:

1. Heat 1 tablespoon of olive oil in a large pan over medium heat. Add the sliced mushrooms and sauté until they are soft and browned. Remove from the pan and set aside.

2. In the same pan, add the remaining olive oil and the finely chopped onion. Sauté until the onion is translucent.

3. Add the minced garlic and Arborio rice, stirring to coat the rice with the oil, and toast it slightly for about 2 minutes.

4. If using, pour in the white wine and stir until it is mostly absorbed by the rice.

5. Begin adding the warm vegetable broth, one ladle at a time, stirring frequently. Wait until each addition is almost fully absorbed before adding the next ladle of broth.

6. Halfway through, add the sautéed mushrooms back into the pan. Continue adding broth and stirring until the rice is creamy and just tender, about 18-20 minutes.

7. Stir in the grated Parmesan cheese, and season with salt and pepper to taste.

8. Serve the mushroom risotto garnished with fresh parsley.

Spinach and Ricotta Stuffed Portobello Mushrooms

Ingredients:

- 4 large Portobello mushroom caps, stems removed
- 1 cup ricotta cheese
- 1 cup fresh spinach, chopped
- 1/4 cup grated Parmesan cheese
- 1 clove garlic, minced
- Salt and pepper to taste
- 2 tablespoons olive oil
- Breadcrumbs for topping (optional)

Instructions:

1. Preheat your oven to 375°F (190°C). Line a baking sheet with parchment paper.
2. Gently clean the Portobello mushrooms with a damp cloth and place them on the prepared baking sheet, gill side up.
3. In a bowl, mix the ricotta cheese, chopped spinach, grated Parmesan cheese, and minced garlic. Season the mixture with salt and pepper.
4. Divide the ricotta and spinach mixture among the mushroom caps, spreading it evenly over the gills.

5. Drizzle olive oil over the stuffed mushrooms and sprinkle breadcrumbs on top if desired for added crunch.

6. Bake in the preheated oven for about 20 minutes, or until the mushrooms are tender and the filling is heated through.

7. Serve the spinach and ricotta stuffed Portobello mushrooms hot.

Tomato Basil Pasta with Grilled Chicken

Ingredients:

- 2 boneless, skinless chicken breasts
- Salt and pepper to taste
- 2 tablespoons olive oil, divided
- 8 ounces whole wheat pasta (spaghetti, penne, or your choice)
- 2 cloves garlic, minced
- 1 can (14 oz) diced tomatoes, undrained
- Fresh basil leaves, chopped (reserve some for garnish)
- Grated Parmesan cheese, for serving

Instructions:

1. Season the chicken breasts with salt and pepper. Heat 1 tablespoon of olive oil in a grill pan over medium-high heat. Grill the chicken for 6-7 minutes on each side, or until fully cooked and juices run clear. Let it rest for a few minutes, then slice thinly.

2. Cook the pasta according to package instructions in salted boiling water until al dente. Drain and set aside.

3. In the same pot, heat the remaining olive oil over medium heat. Add the minced garlic and sauté until fragrant, about 1 minute.

4. Stir in the diced tomatoes with their juice and bring to a simmer. Cook for 5-10 minutes until the sauce thickens slightly.

5. Toss the cooked pasta with the tomato sauce. Add the chopped basil and mix well.

6. Serve the pasta with sliced grilled chicken on top. Garnish with fresh basil leaves and grated Parmesan cheese.

Ratatouille with Baked Polenta

Ingredients for Ratatouille:

- 1 eggplant, diced
- 2 zucchinis, diced
- 1 yellow squash, diced
- 1 red bell pepper, diced
- 1 onion, diced
- 2 cloves garlic, minced
- 1 can (14 oz) diced tomatoes
- 2 tablespoons olive oil
- Salt and pepper to taste
- Fresh thyme and basil, chopped

Ingredients for Polenta:

- 1 cup polenta (cornmeal)
- 4 cups water or vegetable broth
- Salt to taste
- 2 tablespoons butter (optional)
- 1/4 cup grated Parmesan cheese (optional)

Instructions for Ratatouille:

1. Preheat the oven to 375°F (190°C).
2. In a large baking dish, combine the diced eggplant, zucchini, yellow squash, bell pepper, and onion.
3. Add the minced garlic, and diced tomatoes with their juice, olive oil, salt, and pepper. Toss to coat the vegetables evenly.
4. Bake in the preheated oven for 35-40 minutes, stirring occasionally, until the vegetables are tender and lightly caramelized.
5. Stir in the chopped thyme and basil before serving.

Instructions for Polenta:

1. Bring water or vegetable broth to a boil in a large saucepan. Add salt.
2. Gradually whisk in the polenta, reduce the heat to low, and cook, stirring frequently, until the polenta thickens and pulls away from the sides of the pan, about 20-30 minutes.

3. Stir in the butter and Parmesan cheese (if using) until well incorporated.

4. Pour the cooked polenta into a greased baking dish, spreading it into an even layer. Bake at 375°F (190°C) for about 15-20 minutes or until the top is slightly golden.

5. Serve the baked polenta sliced with the ratatouille on top.

Butternut Squash and Kale Stir-Fry

Ingredients:

- 1 medium butternut squash, peeled, seeded, and cut into 1/2-inch cubes
- 1 bunch kale, stems removed and leaves chopped
- 2 tablespoons olive oil
- 3 cloves garlic, minced
- 1 teaspoon ground cumin
- Salt and pepper to taste
- Red pepper flakes (optional, for heat)
- 2 tablespoons water or vegetable broth
- Toasted sesame seeds or chopped nuts for garnish (optional)

Instructions:

1. Heat olive oil in a large skillet or wok over medium heat. Add the minced garlic and sauté until fragrant, about 1 minute.

2. Add the cubed butternut squash to the skillet. Sprinkle with ground cumin, salt, pepper, and red pepper flakes if using. Stir to coat the squash in the seasoning.

3. Cook the butternut squash for about 10 minutes, stirring occasionally, until it starts to soften.

4. Add the chopped kale to the skillet along with 2 tablespoons of water or vegetable broth to help steam the kale.

5. Continue to cook, stirring frequently, until the kale has wilted and the butternut squash is tender but not mushy about 5-7 more minutes.

6. Adjust the seasoning as needed. Serve the stir-fry garnished with toasted sesame seeds or chopped nuts if desired.

Eggplant Parmesan

Ingredients:

- 2 large eggplants, sliced into 1/2-inch rounds
- Salt
- 2 cups marinara sauce
- 2 cups shredded mozzarella cheese
- 1/2 cup grated Parmesan cheese
- 1 cup all-purpose flour (for dredging)
- 2 large eggs, beaten
- 2 cups breadcrumbs
- Olive oil for frying

- Fresh basil leaves for garnish

Instructions:

1. Lay the eggplant slices on paper towels and sprinkle both sides with salt. Let them sit for about 30 minutes to draw out moisture. Pat the slices dry with paper towels.

2. Preheat your oven to 375°F (190°C). Spread a layer of marinara sauce on the bottom of a baking dish.

3. Set up a breading station with three shallow dishes: one with flour, one with beaten eggs, and one with breadcrumbs.

4. Dredge each eggplant slice in flour, dip in the beaten eggs, and then coat with breadcrumbs.

5. Heat olive oil in a large skillet over medium-high heat. Fry the breaded eggplant slices in batches until golden brown on both sides. Transfer to a paper towel-lined plate to drain.

6. Arrange a layer of fried eggplant slices over the sauce in the baking dish. Top with a portion of the marinara sauce, followed by mozzarella and Parmesan cheese. Repeat the layers until all ingredients are used, finishing with cheese on top.

7. Bake in the preheated oven for 25-30 minutes, or until the cheese is bubbly and golden.

8. Garnish with fresh basil leaves before serving. Enjoy this classic Eggplant Parmesan as a hearty and flavorful main dish.

Seared Scallops with Quinoa Salad

Ingredients for Seared Scallops:

- 12 large sea scallops, patted dry
- Salt and pepper to taste
- 1 tablespoon olive oil

Ingredients for Quinoa Salad:

- 1 cup quinoa, rinsed
- 2 cups water or vegetable broth
- 1 cucumber, diced
- 1 bell pepper, diced
- 1/4 cup red onion, finely chopped
- 1/4 cup fresh parsley, chopped
- 2 tablespoons lemon juice
- 2 tablespoons olive oil
- Salt and pepper to taste

Instructions:

1. Cook the quinoa in water or vegetable broth according to package instructions. Fluff with a fork and let cool.
2. In a large bowl, combine the cooled quinoa, cucumber, bell pepper, red onion, and parsley.

3. Dress the quinoa salad with lemon juice, olive oil, salt, and pepper. Toss well and set aside.

4. Season the scallops with salt and pepper. Heat olive oil in a non-stick skillet over high heat.

5. Sear the scallops for about 1-2 minutes on each side, or until they have a golden crust and are just cooked through.

6. Serve the seared scallops over the quinoa salad.

Lentil and Sweet Potato Shepherd's Pie

Ingredients:

- 1 cup dried green lentils, rinsed
- 2 sweet potatoes, peeled and cubed
- 1 tablespoon olive oil
- 1 onion, diced
- 2 carrots, diced
- 2 cloves garlic, minced
- 1 teaspoon dried thyme
- 1/2 teaspoon dried rosemary
- 2 tablespoons tomato paste
- 1 cup vegetable broth
- Salt and pepper to taste
- 1/4 cup milk (or non-dairy alternative)
- 2 tablespoons butter (or non-dairy alternative)

Instructions:

1. Cook the lentils in boiling water until tender, about 20-25 minutes. Drain and set aside.
2. Boil the sweet potatoes until tender. Mash with milk and butter, season with salt and pepper, and set aside.
3. Heat olive oil in a pan. Sauté onion, carrots, and garlic until softened. Add thyme, rosemary, and tomato paste; cook for 1 minute.
4. Add cooked lentils and vegetable broth to the pan. Simmer until the mixture thickens. Season with salt and pepper.
5. Transfer the lentil mixture to a baking dish. Top with the mashed sweet potatoes.
6. Bake at 375°F (190°C) for 20-25 minutes, or until the top is slightly golden.
7. Serve warm.

Zucchini Lasagna

Ingredients:

- 4 large zucchinis, sliced lengthwise into thin strips
- Salt
- 1 pound ground turkey or a vegetarian ground meat alternative
- 1 onion, chopped
- 2 cloves garlic, minced

- 1 can (28 oz) crushed tomatoes
- 1 teaspoon dried oregano
- 1 teaspoon dried basil
- 1 cup ricotta cheese
- 1 egg
- 1/4 cup grated Parmesan cheese
- 2 cups shredded mozzarella cheese

Instructions:

1. Lay zucchini slices on paper towels, sprinkle with salt and let sit for 15 minutes to draw out moisture. Pat dry.
2. Brown the ground turkey with onion and garlic in a pan. Add crushed tomatoes, oregano, and basil. Simmer for 20 minutes.
3. Mix ricotta cheese with egg and Parmesan.
4. In a baking dish, layer zucchini strips, ricotta mixture, meat sauce, and mozzarella. Repeat layers.
5. Bake at 375°F (190°C) for 50 minutes. Let stand for 10 minutes before serving.

Carrot and Celery Sticks with Hummus

Ingredients:

- 2 large carrots, peeled
- 2 stalks of celery
- 1 cup hummus (store-bought or homemade)

Instructions:

1. Wash the carrots and celery thoroughly under cold water.
2. Cut the carrots and celery into sticks approximately 3-4 inches long and 1/2 inch wide.
3. Arrange the carrot and celery sticks on a serving plate.
4. Place the hummus in a small bowl in the center of the plate for easy dipping.
5. Serve the carrot and celery sticks with hummus.

Cucumber Salad with Yogurt and Dill Dressing

Ingredients for Salad:

- 2 medium cucumbers, thinly sliced
- 1/4 red onion, thinly sliced (optional)

Ingredients for Dressing:

- 1 cup plain low-fat Greek yogurt
- 2 tablespoons fresh dill, chopped
- 1 tablespoon lemon juice
- 1 garlic clove, minced
- Salt and pepper to taste

Instructions:

1. In a serving bowl, combine the thinly sliced cucumbers and red onion (if using).
2. In a separate small bowl, whisk together the Greek yogurt, chopped dill, lemon juice, and minced garlic to create the dressing. Season with salt and pepper to taste.
3. Pour the yogurt and dill dressing over the cucumber slices and gently toss to ensure all the slices are evenly coated.
4. Chill the cucumber salad in the refrigerator for about 30 minutes before serving to allow the flavors to meld.
5. Serve the cucumber salad.

Baked Sweet Potato Fries

Ingredients:

- 2 large sweet potatoes, peeled
- 2 tablespoons olive oil

- Salt and pepper to taste
- 1/2 teaspoon paprika (optional for added flavor)
- Fresh parsley, chopped for garnish (optional)

Instructions:

1. Preheat your oven to 425°F (220°C). Line a baking sheet with parchment paper for easy cleanup.
2. Cut the sweet potatoes into sticks about 1/4 inch thick and 3-4 inches long, trying to keep them as uniform as possible for even cooking.
3. In a large bowl, toss the sweet potato sticks with olive oil, salt, pepper, and paprika if using, ensuring all the pieces are evenly coated.
4. Spread the sweet potato fries in a single layer on the prepared baking sheet, making sure they're not touching to ensure they crisp up.
5. Bake in the preheated oven for about 20-25 minutes, turning halfway through the cooking time, until they are golden brown and crispy.
6. Garnish with fresh parsley before serving, if desired.

Cherry Tomatoes Stuffed with Cottage Cheese

Ingredients:

- 12 large cherry tomatoes
- 1/2 cup cottage cheese
- 1 tablespoon fresh herbs (such as chives or parsley), finely chopped
- Salt and pepper to taste
- Fresh basil leaves for garnish (optional)

Instructions:

1. Slice the tops of the cherry tomatoes and use a small spoon or melon baller to carefully scoop out the seeds and insides, creating a hollow space inside each tomato.
2. In a small bowl, mix the cottage cheese with the chopped fresh herbs, salt, and pepper until well combined.
3. Using a small spoon or a piping bag, fill each hollowed-out cherry tomato with the herbed cottage cheese mixture.
4. Place the stuffed cherry tomatoes on a serving platter. Garnish with fresh basil leaves if desired and serve immediately.

Apple Slices with Almond Butter

Ingredients:

- 2 large apples, any variety
- 1/2 cup almond butter
- A sprinkle of cinnamon (optional)

Instructions:

1. Wash the apples thoroughly and pat them dry.
2. Core the apples and slice them into thin rounds or wedges, depending on your preference.
3. Arrange the apple slices on a serving plate or platter.
4. Place the almond butter in a small bowl for easy dipping. If the almond butter is too thick, you can slightly warm it in the microwave for a few seconds to soften.
5. Sprinkle the apple slices with a little cinnamon if desired for added flavor.
6. Serve the apple slices alongside the bowl of almond butter.

Roasted Brussels Sprouts with a Balsamic Glaze

Ingredients:

- 1 pound Brussels sprouts, trimmed and halved
- 2 tablespoons olive oil

- Salt and pepper to taste

- 1/4 cup balsamic vinegar

- 2 tablespoons honey or maple syrup

Instructions:

1. Preheat your oven to 400°F (200°C).

2. In a large bowl, toss the Brussels sprouts with olive oil, salt, and pepper until they are evenly coated.

3. Spread the Brussels sprouts on a baking sheet in a single layer, cut side down.

4. Roast in the preheated oven for about 20-25 minutes, or until they are tender and the edges are caramelized and crispy.

5. While the Brussels sprouts are roasting, prepare the glaze. In a small saucepan, bring the balsamic vinegar and honey (or maple syrup) to a simmer over medium heat. Reduce the heat and let it simmer until the mixture thickens and reduces by about half, stirring occasionally.

6. Once the Brussels sprouts are done, transfer them to a serving dish. Drizzle the balsamic glaze over the roasted Brussels sprouts.

7. Serve the Brussels sprouts warm, garnished with additional salt and pepper if needed.

Kale Chips

Ingredients:

- 1 bunch of kale, washed and dried
- 1 tablespoon olive oil
- Salt to taste
- Optional seasonings: garlic powder, smoked paprika, nutritional yeast

Instructions:

1. Preheat your oven to 300°F (150°C). Line a baking sheet with parchment paper.
2. Remove the stems from the kale and tear the leaves into bite-sized pieces.
3. In a large bowl, toss the kale pieces with olive oil and salt, ensuring each piece is lightly coated. If using, sprinkle your choice of optional seasonings over the kale and toss again.
4. Spread the kale in a single layer on the prepared baking sheet, making sure the pieces don't overlap to ensure they crisp up evenly.
5. Bake in the preheated oven for about 10-15 minutes, or until the edges are slightly browned and the kale is crispy. Keep an eye on them to prevent burning.
6. Let the kale chips cool slightly before serving.

Mixed Berry Fruit Salad

Ingredients:

- 1 cup strawberries, hulled and halved
- 1 cup blueberries
- 1 cup raspberries
- 1 cup blackberries
- 2 tablespoons honey or maple syrup (optional)
- 1 tablespoon fresh lemon juice
- Fresh mint leaves for garnish (optional)

Instructions:

1. Gently rinse the berries and pat them dry with paper towels. Make sure they are fully dry to prevent the salad from becoming soggy.
2. In a large bowl, combine the strawberries, blueberries, raspberries, and blackberries.
3. If using, drizzle honey or maple syrup over the berries for a touch of sweetness. Add the lemon juice to add a bit of zest and to help keep the fruit vibrant.
4. Gently toss the berries with the honey and lemon juice until evenly coated. Be careful not to crush the berries.
5. Refrigerate the fruit salad for about 30 minutes to allow the flavors to meld.

6. Serve the mixed berry fruit salad chilled, garnished with fresh mint leaves if desired.

Rice Cakes Topped with Avocado and Tomato

Ingredients:

- 4 rice cakes

- 1 ripe avocado

- 1 medium tomato, sliced

- Salt and pepper to taste

- Red pepper flakes (optional, for a bit of heat)

- Lemon juice (optional, for a tangy flavor)

- Fresh basil leaves or microgreens for garnish (optional)

Instructions:

1. Peel and pit the avocado. In a small bowl, mash the avocado with a fork until it reaches a creamy consistency. Season with salt, pepper, and a few drops of lemon juice if desired.

2. Spread the mashed avocado evenly over the rice cakes.

3. Arrange the tomato slices on top of the mashed avocado on each rice cake.

4. Season the tomato slices with a pinch of salt, pepper, and red pepper flakes if using.

5. Garnish with fresh basil leaves or microgreens for a fresh touch and added flavor and serve immediately.

Steamed Green Beans with Lemon Zest

Ingredients:

- 1 pound green beans, ends trimmed
- 1 tablespoon olive oil
- Zest of 1 lemon
- Salt and pepper to taste
- Lemon wedges for serving (optional)

Instructions:

1. Steam the green beans until they are tender but still crisp, about 3-5 minutes. You can use a steamer basket over boiling water or a microwave steamer.
2. Once the green beans are steamed, transfer them to a serving bowl.
3. While the green beans are still warm, toss them with olive oil and lemon zest. Season with salt and pepper to taste.
4. Serve the green beans immediately, garnished with additional lemon zest if desired. Offer lemon wedges on the side for guests to add an extra squeeze of lemon juice if they prefer.

CHAPTER 6: Soups and Salads

Carrot Ginger Soup

Ingredients:

- 1 tablespoon olive oil
- 1 onion, chopped
- 2 cloves of garlic, minced
- 2 tablespoons fresh ginger, grated
- 1 pound carrots, peeled and chopped
- 4 cups vegetable broth
- Salt and pepper to taste
- Fresh parsley or cilantro for garnish (optional)

Instructions:

1. Heat the olive oil in a large pot over medium heat. Add the chopped onion and sauté until translucent, about 5 minutes.
2. Add the minced garlic and grated ginger to the pot and cook for another minute, until fragrant.
3. Add the chopped carrots to the pot and stir to combine with the onion, garlic, and ginger.
4. Pour in the vegetable broth and bring the mixture to a boil. Reduce the heat to low and simmer, covered, until the carrots are tender about 20-25 minutes.

5. Once the carrots are soft, use an immersion blender to puree the soup until smooth. Alternatively, you can carefully transfer the soup to a blender to puree in batches.

6. Season the soup with salt and pepper to taste. Adjust the consistency with more vegetable broth or water if necessary.

7. Serve the soup hot, garnished with fresh parsley or cilantro if desired.

Broccoli Almond Soup

Ingredients:

*   1 tablespoon olive oil
*   1 onion, chopped
*   2 cloves of garlic, minced
*   4 cups broccoli florets
*   4 cups vegetable broth
*   1/2 cup almonds, toasted and chopped (plus more for garnish)
*   Salt and pepper to taste
*   A splash of lemon juice (optional)
*   Low-fat cream for garnish (optional)

Instructions:

1. In a large pot, heat the olive oil over medium heat. Add the chopped onion and sauté until it's soft and translucent, about 5 minutes.

2. Add the minced garlic to the pot and cook for another minute until fragrant.

3. Add the broccoli florets to the pot, stirring to combine them with the onion and garlic.

4. Pour in the vegetable broth and bring the mixture to a boil. Once boiling, reduce the heat to low and let it simmer, covered until the broccoli is tender, about 15-20 minutes.

5. Stir in the toasted and chopped almonds, reserving some for garnish.

6. Use an immersion blender to puree the soup until smooth, or transfer the soup to a blender and puree in batches.

7. Season the soup with salt and pepper to taste, and add a splash of lemon juice if using.

8. Serve the soup hot, garnished with a swirl of low-fat cream and the reserved toasted almonds.

Tomato Basil Soup

Ingredients:

- 2 tablespoons olive oil
- 1 onion, finely chopped
- 2 cloves garlic, minced
- 1 can (28 oz) crushed tomatoes
- 4 cups vegetable broth
- 1/4 cup fresh basil leaves, chopped, plus more for garnish

- Salt and pepper to taste

- 1 teaspoon sugar (optional, to balance acidity)

- 2 tablespoons heavy cream or coconut milk (optional, for creaminess)

Instructions:

1. In a large pot, heat the olive oil over medium heat. Add the chopped onion and sauté until translucent, about 5 minutes.

2. Add the minced garlic and cook for an additional minute until fragrant.

3. Pour in the crushed tomatoes and vegetable broth. Stir to combine.

4. Add the chopped basil, salt, pepper, and sugar (if using). Bring the mixture to a boil, then reduce the heat and let it simmer for 20-30 minutes to allow the flavors to meld.

5. Use an immersion blender to puree the soup until smooth, or carefully transfer the soup to a blender and puree in batches.

6. Stir in the heavy cream or coconut milk (if using) for a richer, creamier texture.

7. Adjust the seasoning if necessary. Serve the soup hot, garnished with fresh basil leaves.

Split Pea Soup

Ingredients:

- 1 tablespoon olive oil

- 1 onion, chopped

- 2 carrots, peeled and diced

- 2 stalks celery, diced

- 1 pound dried split peas, rinsed and sorted

- 6 cups vegetable broth or water

- 1 bay leaf

- Salt and pepper to taste

- 1 teaspoon dried thyme (optional)

- 1 teaspoon smoked paprika (optional, for a smoky flavor)

Instructions:

1. In a large pot, heat the olive oil over medium heat. Add the chopped onion, diced carrots, and celery. Sauté until the vegetables are softened, about 5-7 minutes.

2. Add the rinsed split peas to the pot along with the vegetable broth or water, bay leaf, salt, pepper, dried thyme, and smoked paprika (if using).

3. Bring the mixture to a boil, then reduce the heat to low. Cover and simmer for 1 to 1.5 hours, stirring occasionally, until the split peas are completely soft and the soup has thickened.

4. Remove the bay leaf and discard it. Use an immersion blender to partially puree the soup if a smoother texture is desired, leaving some chunks for texture.

5. Adjust the seasoning if necessary. Serve the soup warm, with a crusty piece of bread if desired.

Pumpkin Soup

Ingredients:

- 2 tablespoons olive oil
- 1 onion, chopped
- 2 cloves garlic, minced
- 1 small pumpkin (about 2 pounds), peeled, seeded, and cubed
- 4 cups vegetable broth
- Salt and pepper to taste
- 1 teaspoon ground cinnamon
- 1/2 teaspoon ground nutmeg
- 1 cup coconut milk or heavy cream
- Pumpkin seeds for garnish (optional)

Instructions:

1. In a large pot, heat the olive oil over medium heat. Add the chopped onion and sauté until translucent, about 5 minutes.

2. Add the minced garlic and cook for an additional minute until fragrant.

3. Add the cubed pumpkin to the pot and cook for a few minutes, stirring occasionally.

4. Pour in the vegetable broth and bring the mixture to a boil. Season with salt, pepper, cinnamon, and nutmeg.

5. Reduce the heat to low, cover, and simmer for 20-25 minutes or until the pumpkin is tender and easily pierced with a fork.

6. Use an immersion blender to puree the soup until smooth. Alternatively, carefully transfer the soup to a blender and puree in batches.

7. Stir in the coconut milk or heavy cream, and adjust the seasoning if necessary.

8. Serve the pumpkin soup hot, garnished with pumpkin seeds if desired.

Arugula and Pear Salad

Ingredients:

- 4 cups arugula, washed and dried
- 1 ripe pear, cored and thinly sliced
- 1/4 cup walnuts, toasted and chopped
- 1/4 cup crumbled goat cheese or feta cheese
- 2 tablespoons balsamic vinegar
- 1 tablespoon olive oil
- Salt and pepper to taste
- Honey (optional, for drizzling)

Instructions:

1. In a large salad bowl, combine the arugula and sliced pear.
2. Add the toasted walnuts and crumbled goat cheese or feta to the bowl.
3. In a small bowl, whisk together the balsamic vinegar and olive oil. Season with salt and pepper.
4. Drizzle the dressing over the salad and toss gently to combine.
5. If desired, drizzle a bit of honey over the salad for a touch of sweetness.
6. Serve the salad immediately.

Quinoa Tabbouleh

Ingredients:

- 1 cup quinoa
- 2 cups water
- 1/4 cup olive oil
- 1/4 cup lemon juice
- 2 cups fresh parsley, finely chopped
- 1 cup fresh mint, finely chopped
- 2 tomatoes, diced
- 1 cucumber, diced
- Salt and pepper to taste

Instructions:

1. Rinse the quinoa under cold water until the water runs clear. In a medium saucepan, combine the quinoa and water. Bring to a boil, then reduce heat to low, cover, and simmer for 15 minutes or until the quinoa is tender and the water is absorbed. Fluff with a fork and let cool to room temperature.

2. In a large bowl, whisk together the olive oil and lemon juice. Season with salt and pepper to taste.

3. Add the cooled quinoa to the dressing in the bowl, along with the chopped parsley, mint, tomatoes, and cucumber. Toss well to combine all the ingredients.

4. Adjust the seasoning if necessary and refrigerate for at least 30 minutes to allow the flavors to meld.

5. Serve the quinoa tabbouleh chilled as a refreshing and nutritious side dish or salad.

Beet and Goat Cheese Salad

Ingredients:

- 4 medium beets, roasted, peeled, and sliced
- 1/4 cup balsamic vinegar
- 1/3 cup olive oil
- Salt and pepper to taste
- 4 cups mixed salad greens

- 1/2 cup goat cheese, crumbled

- 1/4 cup walnuts, toasted and chopped

- Fresh basil leaves for garnish (optional)

Instructions:

1. Preheat your oven to 400°F (200°C). Wrap the whole beets in foil and roast them in the oven for about 1 hour or until they are tender when pierced with a fork. Allow them to cool, then peel and slice them.

2. In a small bowl, whisk together the balsamic vinegar and olive oil. Season with salt and pepper to create the dressing.

3. Arrange the mixed salad greens on a serving platter or in individual salad bowls. Top the greens with the sliced roasted beets.

4. Sprinkle the crumbled goat cheese and toasted walnuts over the beets and greens.

5. Drizzle the balsamic dressing over the salad just before serving.

6. Garnish with fresh basil leaves if desired.

Cucumber and Dill Salad

Ingredients:

- 2 large cucumbers, thinly sliced

- 1/4 cup red onion, thinly sliced

- 1/4 cup fresh dill, chopped

- 1/4 cup white vinegar

- 2 tablespoons olive oil

- 1 tablespoon sugar (optional, adjust to taste)

- Salt and pepper to taste

Instructions:

1. In a large bowl, combine the thinly sliced cucumbers, red onion, and chopped dill.

2. In a small bowl or jar, whisk together the white vinegar, olive oil, and sugar (if using) until well combined. Season with salt and pepper to taste.

3. Pour the dressing over the cucumber mixture and toss gently to ensure all the slices are evenly coated with the dressing.

4. Cover and refrigerate the salad for at least 30 minutes to allow the flavors to meld together.

5. Before serving, give the salad a quick toss and adjust the seasoning if necessary.

6. Serve chilled as a refreshing and crisp side dish perfect for any meal.

Mediterranean Chickpea Salad

Ingredients:

- 1 can (15 oz) chickpeas, drained and rinsed

- 1 cup cherry tomatoes, halved

- 1 cucumber, diced

- 1/2 red onion, finely chopped

- 1/2 cup Kalamata olives, pitted and halved

- 1/2 cup feta cheese, crumbled

- 1/4 cup fresh parsley, chopped

- 1/4 cup olive oil

- 2 tablespoons lemon juice

- 1 garlic clove, minced

- 1 teaspoon dried oregano

- Salt and pepper to taste

Instructions:

In a large salad bowl, combine the chickpeas, cherry tomatoes, diced cucumber, chopped red onion, Kalamata olives, crumbled feta cheese, and chopped parsley.

In a small bowl or jar, whisk together the olive oil, lemon juice, minced garlic, dried oregano, salt, and pepper to create the dressing.

Pour the dressing over the salad ingredients in the bowl and toss well to ensure everything is evenly coated with the dressing.

Let the salad sit for about 10-15 minutes before serving to allow the flavors to combine and serve the Mediterranean chickpea salad.

CHAPTER 7: Desserts

Pineapple Sorbet

Ingredients:

- 1 ripe pineapple, peeled, cored, and chopped
- 1/2 cup sugar or honey (adjust according to taste)
- 1 tablespoon lime juice

Instructions:

1. Place the chopped pineapple in a blender or food processor. Add the sugar or honey and lime juice.
2. Blend the mixture until smooth. Taste and adjust the sweetness if necessary.
3. Pour the pineapple mixture into a shallow baking dish or a freezer-safe container.
4. Freeze for about 2 hours, or until the mixture starts to solidify around the edges.
5. Remove from the freezer and stir well, breaking up any frozen sections. Return to the freezer.
6. Repeat the stirring process every 30 minutes for about 2-3 hours, until the sorbet is fully frozen but still somewhat soft for scooping.

7. Serve the pineapple sorbet in chilled bowls or glasses. Optionally, garnish with a sprig of mint or a slice of lime for a refreshing touch.

Peach and Almond Crisp

Ingredients for the Filling:

- 4-5 ripe peaches, peeled and sliced
- 2 tablespoons sugar or honey
- 1 tablespoon cornstarch
- 1 teaspoon vanilla extract
- 1/2 teaspoon ground cinnamon

Ingredients for the Topping:

- 1/2 cup rolled oats
- 1/2 cup almond flour
- 1/4 cup sliced almonds
- 1/4 cup brown sugar or coconut sugar
- 1/4 cup unsalted butter, melted (or coconut oil for a dairy-free option)
- Pinch of salt

Instructions:

1. Preheat the oven to 375°F (190°C). Grease a baking dish with a bit of butter or cooking spray.

2. In a large bowl, combine the sliced peaches, sugar or honey, cornstarch, vanilla extract, and cinnamon. Toss gently until the peaches are evenly coated. Transfer the peach mixture to the prepared baking dish.

3. In another bowl, mix the rolled oats, almond flour, sliced almonds, brown sugar, melted butter, and a pinch of salt until the mixture resembles coarse crumbs.

4. Evenly sprinkle the oat and almond topping over the peach filling.

5. Bake in the preheated oven for 30-35 minutes, or until the topping is golden brown and the peach filling is bubbling.

6. Allow the peach and almond crisp to cool slightly before serving. Enjoy warm, optionally with a dollop of low-fat Greek yogurt or a scoop of dairy-free vanilla ice cream on top.

Carrot and Walnut Cake

Ingredients:

- 2 cups grated carrots
- 1 cup whole wheat flour
- 1/2 cup almond flour
- 1 teaspoon baking soda
- 1/2 teaspoon salt
- 1 teaspoon cinnamon
- 1/2 cup unsweetened applesauce

- 1/4 cup olive oil or melted coconut oil

- 1/2 cup honey or maple syrup

- 2 eggs

- 1 teaspoon vanilla extract

- 1/2 cup walnuts, chopped

- Optional: Cream cheese frosting (use low-fat cream cheese for a lighter option)

Instructions:

1. Preheat your oven to 350°F (175°C). Grease and flour a 9-inch cake pan.

2. In a large bowl, mix the whole wheat flour, almond flour, baking soda, salt, and cinnamon.

3. In a separate bowl, whisk together the applesauce, oil, honey or maple syrup, eggs, and vanilla extract until well combined.

4. Add the wet ingredients to the dry ingredients and stir until just combined. Fold in the grated carrots and chopped walnuts.

5. Pour the batter into the prepared cake pan and smooth the top.

6. Bake for 25-30 minutes, or until a toothpick inserted into the center comes out clean.

7. Let the cake cool in the pan for 10 minutes, then transfer to a wire rack to cool completely.

8. If desired, frost the cake with cream cheese frosting once it's completely cooled. Garnish with additional chopped walnuts.

Cherry Almond Clafoutis

Ingredients:

- 1 tablespoon unsalted butter, for greasing
- 2 cups fresh cherries, pitted
- 3 eggs
- 1 cup almond milk (or any milk of choice)
- 1/2 cup granulated sugar or honey
- 1 teaspoon almond extract
- 1/2 cup all-purpose flour (or almond flour for a gluten-free option)
- 1/4 teaspoon salt
- Powdered sugar for dusting (optional)
- Sliced almonds for garnish (optional)

Instructions:

1. Preheat your oven to 375°F (190°C). Grease a 9-inch pie dish or cast-iron skillet with butter.
2. Scatter the pitted cherries evenly over the bottom of the greased dish.
3. In a blender, combine the eggs, almond milk, sugar or honey, almond extract, flour, and salt. Blend until the mixture is smooth.
4. Pour the batter over the cherries in the dish.

5. Bake for 35-40 minutes, or until the clafoutis is puffed and golden brown and a toothpick inserted into the center comes out clean.

6. Let the clafoutis cool slightly before dusting with powdered sugar and garnishing with sliced almonds if desired.

7. Serve the cherry almond clafoutis warm or at room temperature as a delightful dessert or brunch dish.

Coconut Mango Mousse

Ingredients:

- 2 ripe mangoes, peeled and chopped (reserve some pieces for garnish)
- 1 can (13.5 oz) full-fat coconut milk, chilled overnight
- 2 tablespoons honey or maple syrup, adjust to taste
- 1 teaspoon vanilla extract
- Fresh mint leaves for garnish (optional)

Instructions:

1. Place the chopped mangoes in a blender or food processor and puree until smooth. Set aside a few tablespoons of the puree for garnish.

2. Open the chilled can of coconut milk and scoop out the solid coconut cream into a mixing bowl, leaving the liquid behind.

3. Using an electric mixer, whip the coconut cream until it forms soft peaks.

4. Gently fold the mango puree, honey (or maple syrup), and vanilla extract into the whipped coconut cream until well combined.

5. Spoon the mousse into serving dishes or glasses. Chill in the refrigerator for at least 1 hour to set.

6. Before serving, garnish each mousse with a spoonful of the reserved mango puree and fresh mint leaves if desired.

Grilled Peaches with Honey

Ingredients:

- 4 ripe peaches, halved and pitted
- 2 tablespoons olive oil or melted butter
- 4 tablespoons honey
- Ground cinnamon for sprinkling
- Vanilla ice cream or Greek yogurt for serving (optional)
- Fresh mint leaves for garnish (optional)

Instructions:

1. Preheat your grill to medium-high heat.

2. Brush the cut sides of the peach halves with olive oil or melted butter.

3. Place the peaches on the grill, cut side down, and grill for about 4-5 minutes or until they have nice grill marks.

4. Flip the peaches over and drizzle each half with honey. Sprinkle with a little ground cinnamon.

5. Grill for an additional 3-4 minutes or until the peaches are tender and caramelized.

6. Serve the grilled peaches warm with a scoop of vanilla ice cream or a dollop of Greek yogurt on top if desired.

7. Garnish with fresh mint leaves before serving for an added touch of freshness.

Poached Pears in Spiced Tea

Ingredients:

- 4 firm but ripe pears, peeled, halved, and cored
- 4 cups water
- 2 black tea bags
- 1/2 cup sugar
- 1 cinnamon stick
- 1 vanilla bean, split lengthwise (or 1 teaspoon vanilla extract)
- 4 cloves
- 1-star anise
- Zest of 1 orange

Instructions:

1. In a large saucepan, bring the water to a boil. Add the tea bags and let them steep for 5 minutes. Remove and discard the tea bags.

2. Add the sugar, cinnamon stick, vanilla bean (or vanilla extract), cloves, star anise, and orange zest to the tea. Stir until the sugar is dissolved.

3. Add the pear halves to the saucepan. Reduce the heat to low, cover, and simmer gently for 15-20 minutes, or until the pears are tender but still hold their shape.

4. Carefully remove the pears from the liquid and set them aside to cool. Increase the heat and boil the remaining liquid until it reduces by half and thickens slightly, forming a syrup.

5. Serve the poached pears drizzled with the spiced tea syrup. Optional: Garnish with a dollop of whipped cream or Greek yogurt and a sprinkle of cinnamon.

Fig and Ricotta Tartlets

Ingredients:

- 1 package (about 1.9 oz) of mini tart shells, pre-baked
- 1 cup ricotta cheese
- 2 tablespoons honey, plus extra for drizzling
- 1/2 teaspoon vanilla extract

- 6-8 fresh figs, sliced

- Chopped pistachios or almonds for garnish (optional)

Instructions:

1. In a mixing bowl, combine the ricotta cheese, 2 tablespoons of honey, and vanilla extract. Stir until the mixture is smooth and creamy.

2. Spoon or pipe the ricotta mixture into the mini tart shells, filling them almost to the top.

3. Arrange the sliced figs on top of the ricotta filling in each tartlet.

4. Drizzle a little extra honey over the figs for added sweetness.

5. Garnish the tartlets with chopped pistachios or almonds if desired for a bit of crunch.

6. Chill the tartlets in the refrigerator for at least 30 minutes before serving. Enjoy these elegant and delicious fig and ricotta tartlets as a delightful dessert or sophisticated snack.

Vanilla and Berry Chia Pudding

Ingredients:

- 1/4 cup chia seeds

- 1 cup almond milk (or any other preferred non-dairy milk)

- 1 tablespoon honey or maple syrup (adjust to taste)

- 1 teaspoon vanilla extract

- 1/2 cup mixed berries (strawberries, blueberries, raspberries, etc.), plus extra for garnish

Instructions:

1. In a mixing bowl, combine the chia seeds, almond milk, honey (or maple syrup), and vanilla extract. Stir well to ensure the chia seeds are fully immersed and start to absorb the liquid.
2. Cover the bowl and refrigerate for at least 2 hours, or overnight, until the mixture thickens and achieves a pudding-like consistency.
3. Before serving, give the chia pudding a good stir to break up any clumps. If the pudding is too thick, you can add a little more almond milk to adjust the consistency.
4. Layer the chia pudding with mixed berries in serving glasses or bowls.
5. Garnish with additional berries on top. Serve chilled as a refreshing and nutritious dessert or breakfast option.

Baked Bananas with Cinnamon and Honey

Ingredients:

- 4 ripe bananas, peeled
- 2 tablespoons honey
- 1/2 teaspoon ground cinnamon

- A pinch of nutmeg (optional)
- 1/4 cup chopped nuts (walnuts, pecans, or almonds), for garnish (optional)
- Vanilla ice cream or Greek yogurt, for serving (optional)

Instructions:

1. Preheat your oven to 350°F (175°C). Line a baking sheet with parchment paper.
2. Slice the bananas in half lengthwise and place them cut-side up on the prepared baking sheet.
3. Drizzle the honey evenly over the banana halves. Sprinkle with ground cinnamon and a pinch of nutmeg if using.
4. Bake in the preheated oven for 12-15 minutes, or until the bananas are soft and caramelized.
5. Remove from the oven and let cool slightly.
6. Serve the baked bananas warm, garnished with chopped nuts if desired. For an indulgent treat, pair with a scoop of vanilla ice cream or a dollop of Greek yogurt.

CONCLUSION

In conclusion, this gout diet cookbook for seniors has been meticulously curated to offer a variety of nutritious, delicious, and gout-friendly recipes that cater specifically to the dietary needs and preferences of older adults managing gout. Each recipe has been selected to reduce purine intake, thereby helping to manage uric acid levels and reduce the risk of gout flare-ups. From comforting soups and vibrant salads to hearty main dishes and delectable desserts, this cookbook provides a comprehensive guide to eating well while navigating the challenges of gout.

It's important to remember that diet is just one aspect of managing gout. Regular exercise, maintaining a healthy weight, staying hydrated, and following your healthcare provider's advice are all critical components of a holistic approach to gout management. By incorporating these recipes into your daily meals, you can enjoy a diverse and satisfying diet that not only caters to your taste buds but also supports your health and well-being.

We hope this cookbook serves as a valuable resource in your journey toward a balanced and gout-friendly diet. Remember, eating well doesn't have to be a compromise on flavor or enjoyment; with the right ingredients and a bit of creativity, every meal can be a delightful experience that nourishes both the body and soul.

28-DAY MEAL PLAN

Day 1:

Breakfast: Banana and Walnut Smoothie

Lunch: Grilled Chicken Salad with Mixed Greens

Dinner: Baked Cod with Lemon and Herbs

Snack: Carrot and Celery Sticks with Hummus

Dessert: Pineapple Sorbet

Day 2:

Breakfast: Avocado Toast on Whole Grain Bread

Lunch: Quinoa and Black Bean Stuffed Peppers

Dinner: Stuffed Acorn Squash

Snack: Apple Slices with Almond Butter

Dessert: Peach and Almond Crisp

Day 3:

Breakfast: Quinoa Breakfast Bowl

Lunch: Lentil Soup with Carrots and Celery

Dinner: Grilled Vegetable Platter

Snack: Kale Chips

Dessert: Carrot and Walnut Cake

Day 4:

Breakfast: Apple Cinnamon Porridge

Lunch: Turkey and Avocado Wrap

Dinner: Lemon Garlic Shrimp and Asparagus

Snack: Mixed Berry Fruit Salad

Dessert: Cherry Almond Clafoutis

Day 5:

Breakfast: Vegetable Omelet

Lunch: Roasted Beet and Goat Cheese Salad

Dinner: Roasted Chicken with Root Vegetables

Snack: Cucumber Salad with Yogurt and Dill Dressing

Dessert: Coconut Mango Mousse

Day 6:

Breakfast: Whole Wheat Pancakes with Maple Syrup

Lunch: Tofu Stir-Fry with Broccoli and Bell Peppers

Dinner: Vegetarian Chili

Snack: Baked Sweet Potato Fries

Dessert: Grilled Peaches with Honey

Day 7:

Breakfast: Chia Seed Pudding with Kiwi

Lunch: Egg Salad on Whole Grain Bread

Dinner: Mushroom Risotto

Snack: Steamed Green Beans with Lemon Zest

Dessert: Poached Pears in Spiced Tea

Day 8:

Breakfast: Cottage Cheese with Pineapple

Lunch: Vegetable and Chickpea Curry

Dinner: Ratatouille with Baked Polenta

Snack: Rice Cakes Topped with Avocado and Tomato

Dessert: Fig and Ricotta Tartlets

Day 9:

Breakfast: Pear and Ginger Muffins

Lunch: Baked Salmon with Dill and Lemon

Dinner: Butternut Squash and Kale Stir-Fry

Snack: Cherry Tomatoes Stuffed with Cottage Cheese

Dessert: Vanilla and Berry Chia Pudding

Day 10:

Breakfast: Veggie Breakfast Wrap

Lunch: Pasta Primavera with Olive Oil and Garlic

Dinner: Eggplant Parmesan

Snack: Roasted Brussels Sprouts with a Balsamic Glaze

Dessert: Baked Bananas with Cinnamon and Honey

Day 11:

Breakfast: Baked Sweet Potato Hash

Lunch: Zucchini Noodles with Tomato and Basil Sauce

Dinner: Seared Scallops with Quinoa Salad

Snack: Cucumber Salad with Yogurt and Dill Dressing

Dessert: Pineapple Sorbet

Day 12:

Breakfast: Avocado Toast on Whole Grain Bread

Lunch: Greek Salad with Chickpeas

Dinner: Lentil and Sweet Potato Shepherd's Pie

Snack: Kale Chips

Dessert: Peach and Almond Crisp

Day 13:

Breakfast: Whole Wheat Pancakes with Maple Syrup

Lunch: Grilled Chicken Salad with Mixed Greens

Dinner: Zucchini Lasagna

Snack: Carrot and Celery Sticks with Hummus

Dessert: Carrot and Walnut Cake

Day 14:

Breakfast: Quinoa Breakfast Bowl

Lunch: Tofu Stir-Fry with Broccoli and Bell Peppers

Dinner: Spinach and Ricotta Stuffed Portobello Mushrooms

Snack: Apple Slices with Almond Butter

Dessert: Cherry Almond Clafoutis

Day 15:

Breakfast: Apple Cinnamon Porridge

Lunch: Roasted Beet and Goat Cheese Salad

Dinner: Grilled Vegetable Platter

Snack: Mixed Berry Fruit Salad

Dessert: Coconut Mango Mousse

Day 16:

Breakfast: Chia Seed Pudding with Kiwi

Lunch: Egg Salad on Whole Grain Bread

Dinner: Mushroom Risotto

Snack: Baked Sweet Potato Fries

Dessert: Grilled Peaches with Honey

Day 17:

Breakfast: Banana and Walnut Smoothie

Lunch: Quinoa and Black Bean Stuffed Peppers

Dinner: Baked Cod with Lemon and Herbs

Snack: Steamed Green Beans with Lemon Zest

Dessert: Poached Pears in Spiced Tea

Day 18:

Breakfast: Veggie Breakfast Wrap

Lunch: Lentil Soup with Carrots and Celery

Dinner: Lemon Garlic Shrimp and Asparagus

Snack: Rice Cakes Topped with Avocado and Tomato

Dessert: Fig and Ricotta Tartlets

Day 19:

Breakfast: Pear and Ginger Muffins

Lunch: Turkey and Avocado Wrap

Dinner: Ratatouille with Baked Polenta

Snack: Cherry Tomatoes Stuffed with Cottage Cheese

Dessert: Vanilla and Berry Chia Pudding

Day 20:

Breakfast: Cottage Cheese with Pineapple

Lunch: Vegetable and Chickpea Curry

Dinner: Butternut Squash and Kale Stir-Fry

Snack: Carrot and Celery Sticks with Hummus

Dessert: Baked Bananas with Cinnamon and Honey

Day 21:

Breakfast: Almond Butter and Banana Sandwich

Lunch: Baked Salmon with Dill and Lemon

Dinner: Eggplant Parmesan

Snack: Kale Chips

Dessert: Pineapple Sorbet

Day 22:

Breakfast: Quinoa Breakfast Bowl

Lunch: Grilled Chicken Salad with Mixed Greens

Dinner: Zucchini Lasagna

Snack: Carrot and Celery Sticks with Hummus

Dessert: Carrot and Walnut Cake

Day 23:

Breakfast: Avocado Toast on Whole Grain Bread

Lunch: Greek Salad with Chickpeas

Dinner: Lentil and Sweet Potato Shepherd's Pie

Snack: Kale Chips

Dessert: Peach and Almond Crisp

Day 24:

Breakfast: Whole Wheat Pancakes with Maple Syrup

Lunch: Tofu Stir-Fry with Broccoli and Bell Peppers

Dinner: Spinach and Ricotta Stuffed Portobello Mushrooms

Snack: Apple Slices with Almond Butter

Dessert: Cherry Almond Clafoutis

Day 25:

Breakfast: Apple Cinnamon Porridge

Lunch: Roasted Beet and Goat Cheese Salad

Dinner: Grilled Vegetable Platter

Snack: Mixed Berry Fruit Salad

Dessert: Coconut Mango Mousse

Day 26:

Breakfast: Chia Seed Pudding with Kiwi

Lunch: Egg Salad on Whole Grain Bread

Dinner: Mushroom Risotto

Snack: Baked Sweet Potato Fries

Dessert: Grilled Peaches with Honey

Day 27:

Breakfast: Banana and Walnut Smoothie

Lunch: Quinoa and Black Bean Stuffed Peppers

Dinner: Baked Cod with Lemon and Herbs

Snack: Steamed Green Beans with Lemon Zest

Dessert: Poached Pears in Spiced Tea

Day 28:

Breakfast: Veggie Breakfast Wrap

Lunch: Lentil Soup with Carrots and Celery

Dinner: Lemon Garlic Shrimp and Asparagus

Snack: Rice Cakes Topped with Avocado and Tomato

www.ingramcontent.com/pod-product-compliance
Lightning Source LLC
Chambersburg PA
CBHW070821260726
48660CB00005B/1941